Ramblings about disinfection

Ramblings about disinfection

By Gaétan Lanthier & Rémi Charlebois

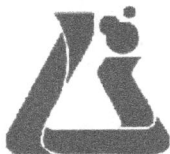

Art Work (book cover): Alex St-Gelais
Translation: Ivan Di Capua, Rémi Charlebois, Gaétan Lanthier

Dépôt légal — Bibliothèque et Archives nationales du Québec, 2016.
Dépôt légal — Bibliothèque et Archives Canada, 2016.

ISBN 978-2-9814674-7-8

Foreword

The cleanliness of our surrounding environment is closely linked to our quality of life. In this book, you will discover, or rediscover, the actions and good practices that contribute to improve our lives in our work environment and beyond.

Among other things, we will address the issues related to infectious risks, product quality, equipment and various aspects or work organisation.

In short, we give you a comprehensive review of the disinfection world of today.

Do not forget to subscribe to our blog:

www.ramblingsaboutdisinfection.com

Best regards,

Gaétan & Rémi

Table of content

Foreword.. 5

Cleaning in Hospitals 7

Romans Used to Say: Automate your Restrooms 15

A Brief History of Bleach.. 17

A Virus Transmitted from Computers to Humans............................... 19

How does UV Disinfection Works? 21

Wipe Out Gastroenteritis!.. 23

Don't be Afraid to Go Micro 25

Hospitals Here and There Around the World.. 27

A Brief History of the Influenza 31

FIFO: First In, First Out also Applies to Disinfectant!........................ 34

Stopping it from Getting Viral 36

MERS-CoV: Practical Tips for Disinfection... 38

Dilution is the Solution 40

How to Reduce Fatigue and Nosocomial Infection at the Same Time 43

Happy Global Handwashing Day 46

Ebola, How to Disinfect Surfaces... 48

Ebola Virus, Are We Ready?... 50

Robots to Destroy Ebola?.. 52

Ebola, How Does it Spread?.. 54

Zika Virus, Where Does It Come From?... 56

Zika Virus is there a Risk for Surface Contamination?........................ 59

Why Choose a Ready-to-use Bleach Based Cleaner-Disinfectant?..................... 61

Ramblings about disinfection – Lalema inc.
Gaétan Lanthier & Rémi Charlebois

Cleaning in Hospitals

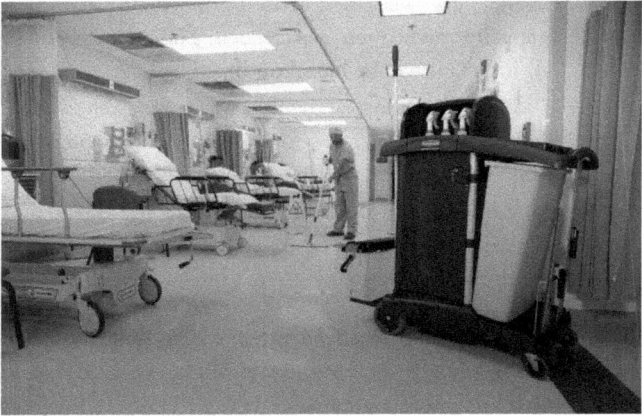

For a long time, cleaning has been all about the look; Fresh smell and the absence of stains or dirt were the criteria to determine that a place is clean. Today, these criteria are still generally accepted in environments such as offices and classrooms.

It is common knowledge, however, that microbes (bacteria or viruses) invisible to the human eye represent a risk for spreading infections. Take the example of the influenza virus: it can survive for up to 48 hours on a hard non-porous surface!

Without cleaning and disinfection procedures or a quality check procedure, microbes can survive in hospital environments. Three key elements have to be considered in order to perform an infective risk analysis:

- Is the patient carrying a disease agent? Disease agents are classified based on their spreading capacity and their virulence. The choice of a disinfectant will be based on this.
- Do the functional activities of a sector represent a risk of spreading infections from the environment? E.g.: food service, offices, Intensive Care, etc.
- The intensity of contact is related to the traffic and the surfaces that are more likely to be touched. E.g.: bathroom fittings.

Have you already performed an infective risk analysis? The next section is going to explain how cleaning allows reducing risks of infection among patients.

Reduce the Risks of Infection Among Patients.

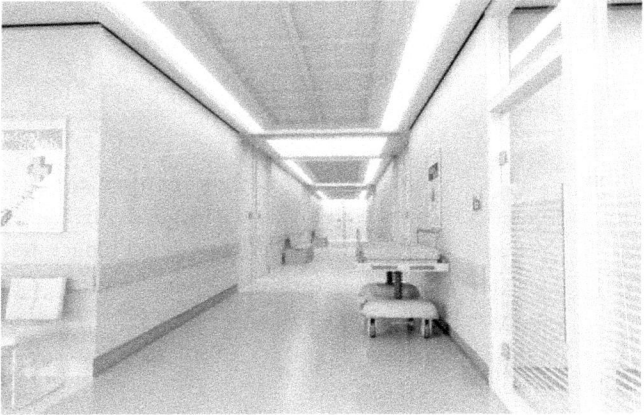

Cleaning in hospitals allows to reduce the risks of infection among patients. This is not the only factor, of course: good personal hygiene habits such as washing hands and the use of protective equipment such as overalls, gloves, masks, or protective glasses are also important elements.

For this reason, interventions must be well coordinated in order to have a good surface maintenance plan. The manager of hygiene and cleanliness should therefore take into account:

- The type of place associated to the level of risk
- The tasks to perform
- The required cleaning frequency

If well applied, a detailed estimate allows validating the cleaning performance.

The global approach is going to be determined by the type of place:

- Regular eradication (e.g.: operating rooms)
- Keeping environmental effects as light as possible (e.g.: low infection risk such as individual office spaces)
- Balance of microorganisms. This approach is based on the competition between good and bad microbes. The presence of good microbes guarantees less space for bad microbes to grow (e.g.: living environments)
- Green cleaning. Approach that uses less toxic products
- Review and improve arrangements and/or surfaces (during conception or renovation)

The next section is going to be about another key factor: the housekeeping staff.

Housekeeping Staff

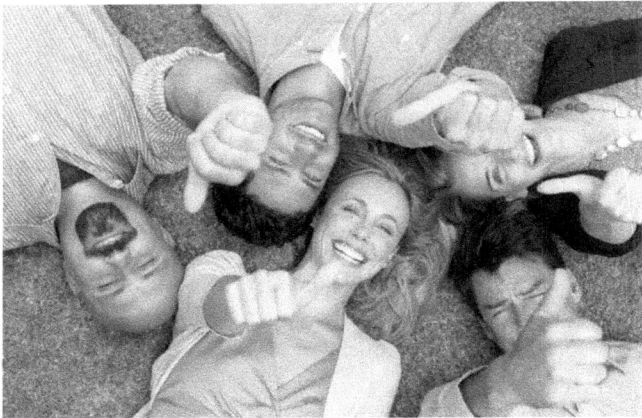

The housekeeping staff represents a key element in the fight against infections in hospital environments. Often little valued, their role in the global strategy of surface cleaning is extremely important.

The hygiene that comes from the work of the cleaning staff requires a high-performance level. In order to reach that, the executing staff and the managers need to master all the different elements representing this profession.

Cleaning products and equipment are undeniably crucial in order to ensure performance during the environment asepsis of any establishment. Therefore, it is important to associate the day-to-day actions of the cleaning staff with a range of products and equipment that favor the quality of their performance.

Since several years, partly due to the devotion and the involvement of many members in the healthcare system, we take into consideration new factors:

- Provincial training
- Establishment of an AEP hygiene and cleanliness in healthcare environments of 630 hours now offered by many school boards
- Provincial day of hygiene and cleanliness
- Etc.

Having said this, the housekeeping staff deserves our deepest gratitude. Thank you so much!

The next section is going to talk more in detail about one aspect of their profession: work organization.

Work Organisation

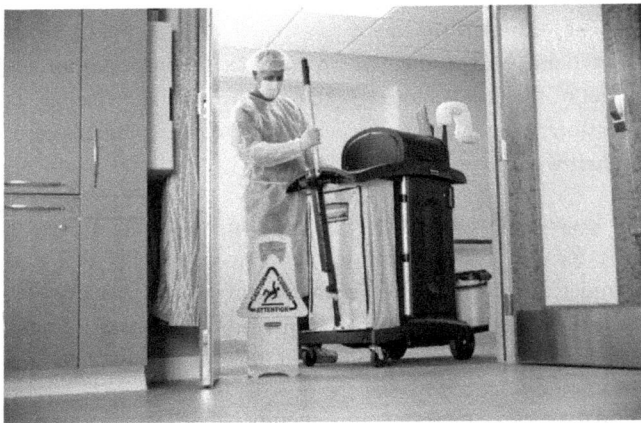

How can proper work organization contribute to the cleanliness of a hospital? How to be in the right place with the right equipment? Here are the questions we are going to answer in this post of the Cleaning in Hospitals series.

Evaluation of production needs

First, we need to assess the needs in hygiene and cleanliness. In order to do this, a standard evaluation is preferable but it needs to be adjusted based on the type of place, units, and traffic.

It is during the evaluation of needs that the hygiene and cleanliness estimate is going to be determined. All daily, weekly, monthly, and annual tasks have to be considered.

Usually, the results are presented by production yields (square meters/hour) or FTE (Full Time Equivalent).

How to reduce time waste

How to measure productivity in a context where an important aspect of the task is moving? Actually, hygiene and cleanliness departments are almost always in the basement, whereas most of their work happens on the floors!

We increase productivity by reducing traveling.

It is for this reason that the cleaning cart needs to be as complete as possible and the water sources or janitor's closets well stocked with supplies (i.e.: paper products or waste bags), equipment, and sanitary products.

Moreover, it is important to remember that a good entrance carpet can greatly reduce dirt.

Have a successful day!

Here are a few hints on how to have a successful day:

- Establish a sequence of actions to perform in a day/week/month
- Define a sequential order of rooms
- Integrate linked and periodical tasks (monthly)
- Make sure to have time gaps to focus on periodical tasks (dusting of high surfaces, polishing, etc.)
- Minimize traveling
- Work by space and not by task
- Distribute tasks equitably
- One look is worth a thousand words: choose a colorful plan together with some graphics instead of a list of tasks on a word file!

Romans Used to Say: Automate your Restrooms

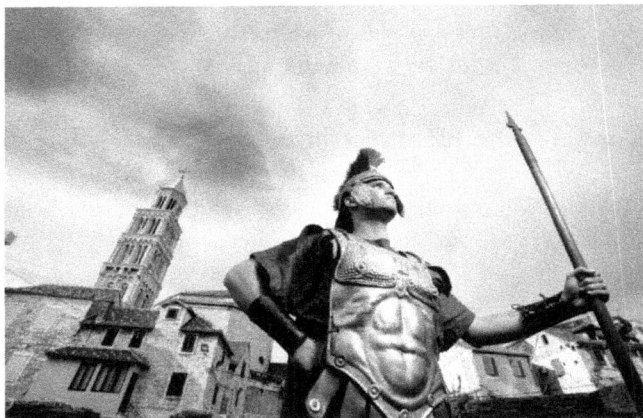

This is not really what the Romans would tell each other after a rough battle against the Gallic, but nowadays the battle is never ending and merciless against the irreducible microbes!

Certain bacteria are good for us

And yet, most of the bacteria are good for us, simply think of yogurts or biological products and you'll see that not all bacteria must be eliminated!

In certain environments such as your home, it's not necessary to eradicate all microbial activity on the surfaces. It's still better to do it in an operating room though!

Let's talk about public restrooms

Whether it is in at clinic, at school, in a shopping mall, a restaurant, or even at the office, certain people are a bit reluctant to touch surfaces. And what about you?

Conceive the ideal restroom

In this ideal restroom, you will find accessories that have been conceived based on 3 fundamental criteria:

- Infection spread risk reduction
- Consumption reduction (environment protection)
- Comfort and well-being of the user

Among these items, you'll find:

- Auto-flush systems
- Continuous cleaning systems
- Auto-faucets
- Automatic doors
- Waterless urinals
- Automatic soap dispensers
- No-touch hand dryers

Ramblings about disinfection – Lalema inc.
Gaétan Lanthier & Rémi Charlebois

A Brief History of Bleach

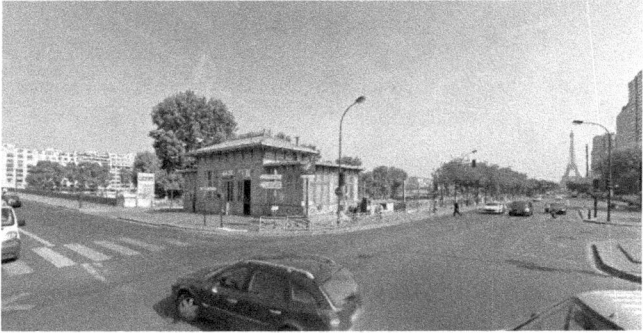

Bleach was studied for the first time by a French chemist named Claude Louis Berthollet in 1775. His factory was based in Paris in the district of… Javel! That is why the French call it: Eau de Javel (Javel water).

At first, bleach was used for laundry and to fade textiles. From 1820, a pharmacist named Antoine Germain Labarraque studied more deeply its disinfecting properties. In the XIX Century, it was commonly used as a disinfectant and water treatment. The NASA used bleach during the Apollo program to disinfect the Apollo XI rocket after its return, in order to avoid contaminating Earth with potential dangerous viruses!

What is Bleach?

Bleach is composed of sodium hypochlorite ($NaClO$). For chemistry fans, its chemical formula is as follows:

$Cl_2 + 2\ NaOH \rightarrow NaCl + NaClO + H_2O.$

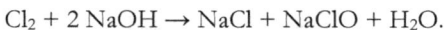

For those who don't like chemistry, well... the formula is the same!

What's new?

Nowadays, bleach is still being used as a disinfectant. Stabilized formulas enable to combine the disinfecting ability of chlorine together with the cleaning ability of surfactants.

Ramblings about disinfection – Lalema inc.
Gaétan Lanthier & Rémi Charlebois

A Virus Transmitted from Computers to Humans

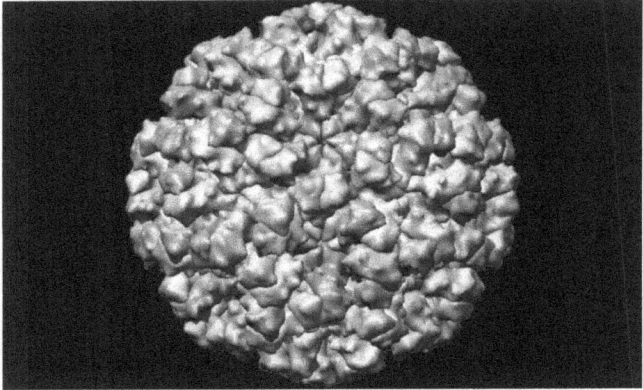

Virus on my keyboard, really?

Did you know that your keyboard and mouse are covered with bacteria and viruses? This may sound obvious when we think about it. Using computers is very common and the risk to be infected seems banal. However, in certain environments such as hospitals, this contamination could reveal critical.

In fact, many bacteria and virus outbreaks have been associated with computers. It's the case for a hospital in Great Britain, where a study revealed that 42% of tested keyboards were contaminated with the MRSA bacteria, which was directly related to higher MRSA infections as compared to other hospitals where keyboard contamination was lower (1). Another study carried out in Great Britain found that keyboards had been a nest for the norovirus, which then lead to a break of gastro-enteritis. A virus transmitted from computers to humans... who would've thought about that!

Don't panic, solutions exist!

First and unforgettable is hand washing. In order to limit bacteria and virus spreads, hand washing is essential. Then, to avoid washing our hands every time we use a computer, an alcohol-based antiseptic liquid would do the trick. If our hands are dirty, washing hands before touching the keyboard is also recommended. Finally, it is wise to disinfect your keyboard and mouse from time to time. A renowned researcher named William Rutala, or Bill for intimates, has demonstrated that computer keyboards do not seem to deteriorate after being cleaned 300 times with different disinfectant solutions.

Long story short, we often forget daily objects as being a breeding ground for viruses and bacteria. For example, mobile phones are often neglected as well despite the fact that we touch them and constantly put them on our face.

But no need to become hypochondriac, it's enough to follow basic preventive measures. In other words, make little changes and set frequent disinfections based on the risk associated with your environment.

How does UV Disinfection Works?

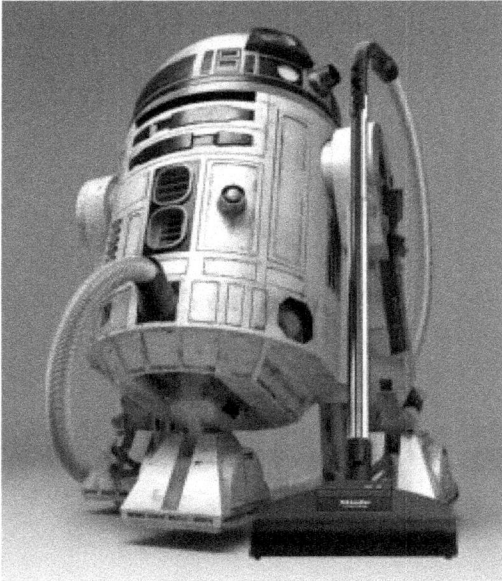

Since 1877, scientists know that microorganisms can be eliminated by UV rays. Nearly 50 years later, however, they discovered the specific type of frequency that was the most damaging.

In the 1950s, researchers knew that UV rays penetrate cells and damage the nucleic acids or deoxyribonucleic acid (DNA) and ribonucleic acid (RNA). This led to the commercial development of multiple UV disinfection devices, primarily with mercury vapor, which produces UV having the most effective frequency for the destruction of microorganisms. Today, UV disinfection devices use xenon UV rays.

UV disinfection is used in many hospitals

UV disinfection devices are used in hospitals such as the ones in Vancouver and Hamilton. It is the natural evolution of the UV disinfection, to which are added the cleaning and disinfecting surface and a good dose of prevention.

Combined with touchless systems for bathrooms and public spaces, hospitals are able to reduce the number of surfaces to be disinfected to prevent nosocomial infections.

In any case, these robots do not replace the housekeeping staff but add a small sector futuristic air ... don't you see a family resemblance with this R2-D2 designed by Agent-Spiff?

Wipe Out Gastroenteritis!

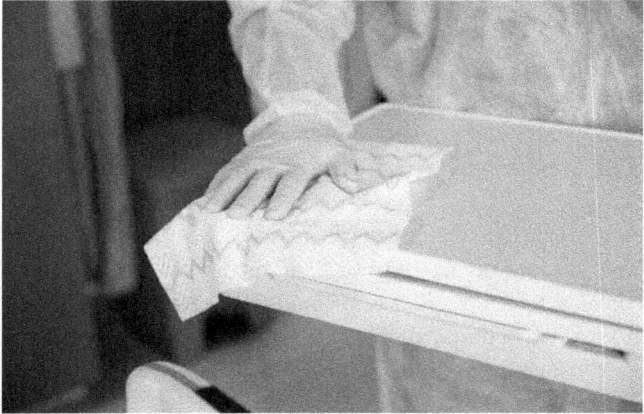

Standard disinfectants are not as effective when facing viruses that cause gastroenteritis.

Approximately 40% of commercial disinfectants that are used to clean surfaces are little or no effective in destroying the norovirus, the virus that causes gastroenteritis. This is what Dr Julie Jean, of the Université de Laval, has found in her recent study. Her research has demonstrated that bleach-based disinfectants are the most effective in reducing the norovirus from surfaces.

The virus that is responsible for gastroenteritis

The norovirus is the main cause of viral gastro-enteritis in health centers. Moreover, it's responsible of half for gastro-enteritis breaks originating from food. This virus spreads mainly through direct contact with the infected people, or indirectly through objects, food, or dirty surfaces.

The effectiveness of disinfectants used for cleaning surfaces is therefore crucial to limit the spread of viruses.

The best strategy to prevent gastroenteritis

As a conclusion, the research suggests that the best strategy to limit the spread of the norovirus is to use a disinfectant containing bleach and leave it in contact with the surface for at least five minutes, ideally ten.

Ramblings about disinfection – Lalema inc.
Gaétan Lanthier & Rémi Charlebois

Don't be Afraid to Go Micro

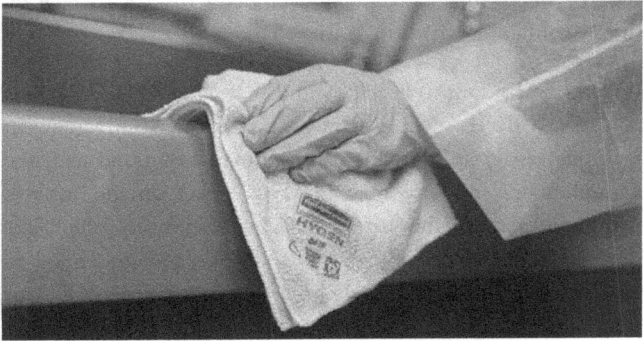

Today it's undeniable that microfibers are superior to cotton fibers. Although the official recommendation of the Ministry of Health and Social Services privileges the use of microfibers, cotton fibers are still pretty common in disinfecting procedures.

What are the differences between cotton and microfibers?

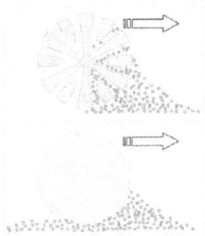

The difference between microfibers and normal fibers are the size of filaments as well as their structure. You can see their superior effectiveness in the image.

It is in fact for this reason that the Ministry of Health and Social Services recommends the use of microfibers for cleaning in hospitals, as their mechanic cleaning ability is greatly increased. Up to 90% of microorganisms can be removed from a surface by simply rubbing it with a microfiber cloth.

It is also important to keep in mind that natural fibers such as cotton can decrease the effectiveness of the disinfectant. In fact, quaternary ammoniums may permanently bond with the natural fibers and lose their ability to react on the surface. Although quats of the 4th and 5th generation are much less sensitive to the type of fiber used, it's still recommended to use synthetic fibers. The same holds for peroxide and oxidant based products such as chlorine; these products may interact with natural fibers. If you don't have access to synthetic fibers, we strongly suggest not soaking your cotton clothes in the disinfecting solution for too long.

Quality of your microfiber cloth!

Beware of microfibers imitations; certain low-quality products won't have the same mechanical effect on surfaces. Also, low quality microfibers often shrink after washing and are more sensitive to hot water and oxidants. At Lalema, our microfiber cloths are all supplied by first choice suppliers. Although a little bit more expensive, these microfiber cloths are more durable and represent the best choice for quality cleaning.

Ramblings about disinfection – Lalema inc.
Gaétan Lanthier & Rémi Charlebois

Hospitals Here and There Around the World

The saying goes, the grass is always greener on the other side of the fence. Let's see what's going on, on the other side!

Sierra Leone

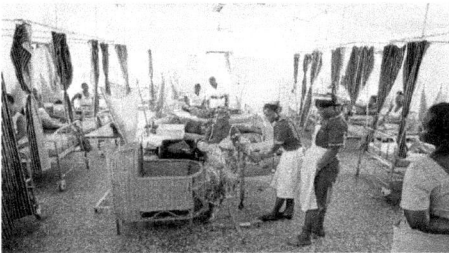

Maternity hospital in Sierra Leone. Since 2010, more and more women are choosing to give birth in hospitals.

Taiwan

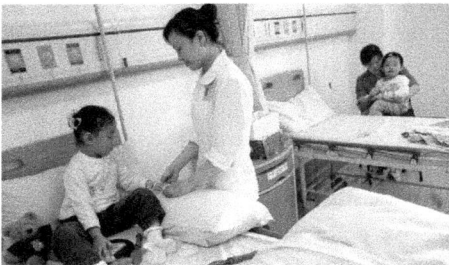

Hospital colors seems to be an international concept!

Sudan

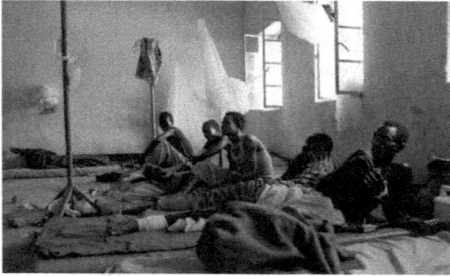

Sometimes budgets do not include beds ...

Russia

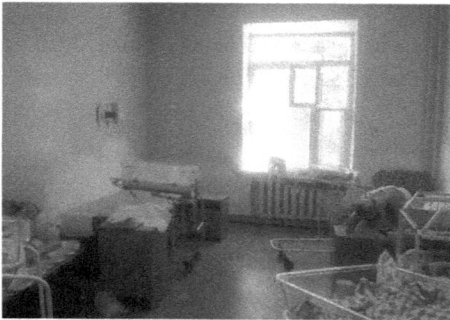

Some Russian hospitals beyond the Urals are still waiting for post-Soviet modernization.

Poland

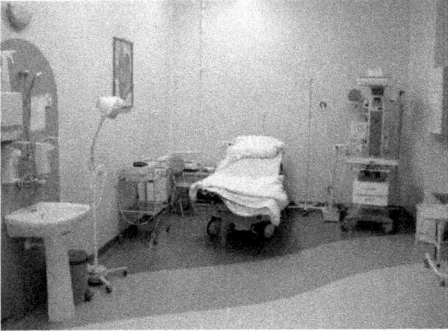

Poland is modernizing its hospitals to override the memories of Soviet rule.

United Arab Emirates

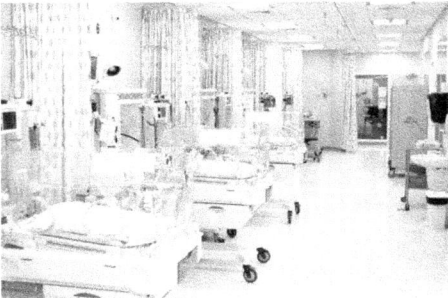

Modern hospitals in Dubai, nothing's too good!

USA

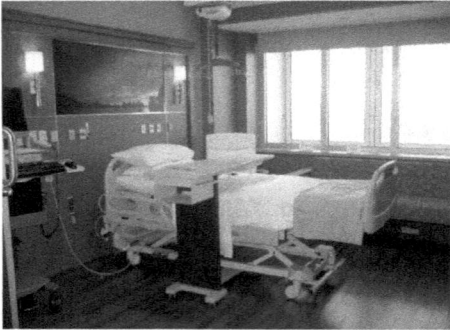

If you have the means, the US private hospitals offer great luxury!

Quebec

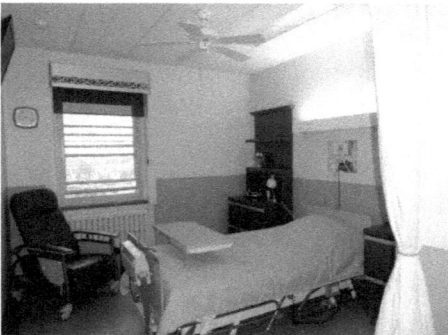

Although hospitals are not all recent or renovated, we can be proud of the quality of care in our hospitals!

A Brief History of the Influenza

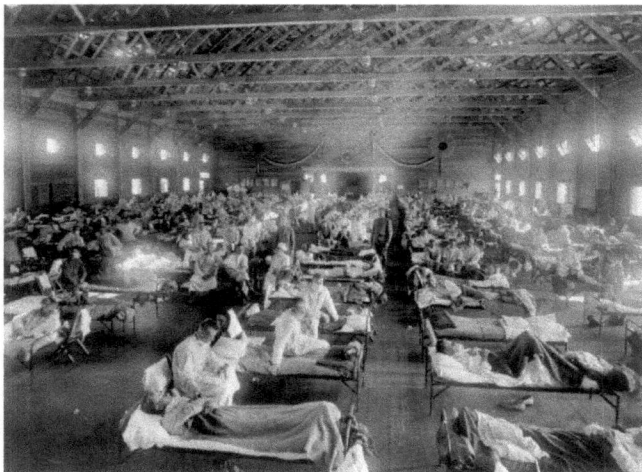

Historical picture of the 1918 Spanish flu at Camp Funston, Kansas, showing the many ill patients.

I would like to talk to you about the Influenza. My mother always told me: "Son, a small flu lasts a week and a big one lasts 7 days." and she was right. Influenza is a respiratory infection that also spreads very easily. It is caused by the influenza virus.

The origin of the flu

Influenza hit human beings in China as early as around - 2500 B.C. With birds, the virus goes back to more than 8000 years ago.

Hippocrates had clearly described Influenza

In -2400, the writings of Hippocrates clearly describe the symptoms of the flu. And since then, history is full of influenza pandemics description. However, before 1850, the data were sometimes difficult to analyze because the symptoms of flu are similar to other diseases such as diphtheria, bubonic plague, typhoid fever and others.

Major known influenza pandemics

Pandemic	Date	Death	Subtype involved	Severity Index
Asian Flu (Russia)	1889–1890	1 million	H2N2 ?	?
Spanish Flu	1918–1920	30 to 100 millions	H1N1	5
Asian Flu	1957–1958	1 to 1,5 millions	H2N2	2
Hong Kong Flu	1968–1969	0,75 to 1 million	H3N2	2
A (H1N1) Flu	2009–2010	18 138	H1N1	

Discovery of the virus

It was long thought that influenza was caused a bacterium. In 1931, the virus was identified in pigs and two years later, in

1933, humans from swab on the throat of a researcher contaminated with the flu.

Discovery of the vaccine

In 1935, we managed to "grow" the virus in embryonated chicken eggs. The first clinical trials between 1936 and 1938 were inconclusive. In 1944, with support from the US Army, we obtained the first effective vaccine based on influenza virus. Research has continued since.

The vaccine in Quebec is available every year in November

Even if you have been vaccinated against the flu last year, you still need to receive it this year. Indeed, antibody levels fall about 6 months after vaccination against influenza, particularly in people whose immune system is weakened.

Preventive measure against the flu

If we cannot escape it, there are still prevention methods:

- Maintain a proper hygiene program (particularly hand washing).
- Get vaccinated.
- Ensure that surfaces are cleaned and disinfected regularly.

FIFO: First In, First Out also Applies to Disinfectant!

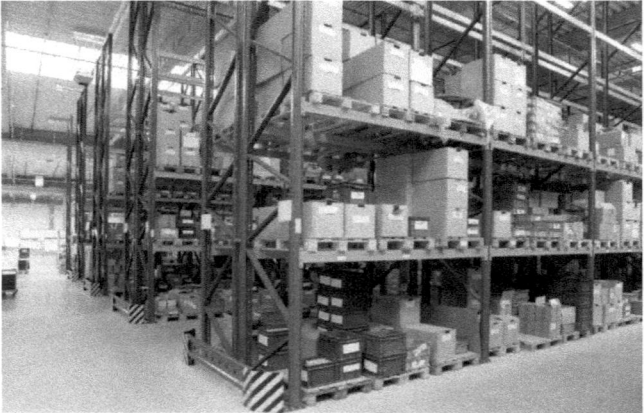

Some of you may be familiar with the FIFO concept. FIFO is a method for organizing and manipulating goods such as food; it is also used in computer science to organize data. In the food industry, FIFO is essential in order to ensure freshness, preventing foodborne illness and controlling costs.

Can a cleaning product expire?

When it comes to disinfectant the same goes, a fresher or let's say a newer product is better. I sometimes hear people saying that soap doesn't expire. Even though the shelf life of soap is way greater than most food items, soaps and other cleaning products do expire.

Same goes for disinfectant the active ingredient of a disinfectant whether it is quats, chlorine or peroxide will diminish over time. Hence to ensure a proper disinfection, it is important to use product that are not expired.

A good way to achieve this is by implementing a FIFO rotation system. By always using the oldest disinfectant that you have in inventory first, you make sure that you won't get stuck with old and maybe expired stuff!

How to know if a cleaning product is expired?

This is a broad question... For disinfectant it is pretty easy, Health Canada and the EPA requires that all disinfectant have an expiration date on their label. Most cleaning products however, do not have an expiration date and the shelf life varies greatly among them.

But some signs won't get you wrong. If the color, the odor, the consistency of the product is changed or if you see a deposit in the product it might be a good sign that the product is expired. In case of doubt, call the manufacturer, with the lot number every good manufacturer will be able to tell you if the product is expired.

Stopping it from Getting Viral

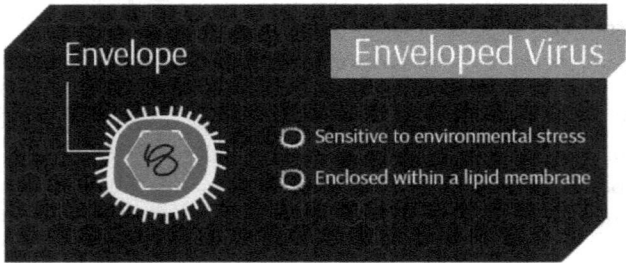

Stopping it from Getting Viral

One disinfecting has to keep in mind what he is trying to get rid of. Disinfectant choice should always consider the microorganism to be eliminated in the environment. Let's remember what we need to consider when disinfecting a virus contaminated environment.

Virology 101

First, let's do a quick recap of what is a virus. A virus is a small infectious agent that can only replicate in another organism. This notion is important, it means that a human virus cannot replicate in food or soil. It is specific to its host. Another important notion about viruses is that they can be either enveloped or not enveloped. The envelope is made of a lipidic barrier originating from the cell the virus replicates in. Regardless of the lipidic membrane virus are made of a protein capsid and genetic material which can either be DNA or RNA.

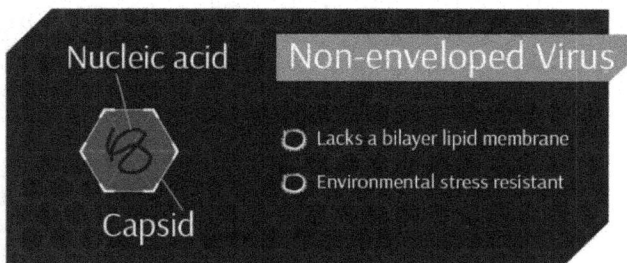

Resistance to disinfectant

Basically, viruses can be divided into two groups regarding their resistance to disinfectant; those are the enveloped and non-enveloped viruses. Non-enveloped viruses are less susceptible to disinfectant. For example, norovirus or hepatitis A agent are small non-enveloped viruses. They are known to be more resistant to environmental stress, such as temperature, UV, low or high humidity levels and disinfectant.

How to disinfect for virus contamination?

First thing first, if your disinfectant has a virucidal claim on the bottle you are fine. You can also look for specific claims, however the general claim is sufficient as it was proven to be effective for multiple viruses. Usually, a minimum of 1,000 ppm of stabilized sodium hypochlorite or 5,000-10,000 ppm of fast acting hydrogen peroxide is a good way to make sure virus in the environment are no more of a threat.

MERS-CoV: Practical Tips for Disinfection

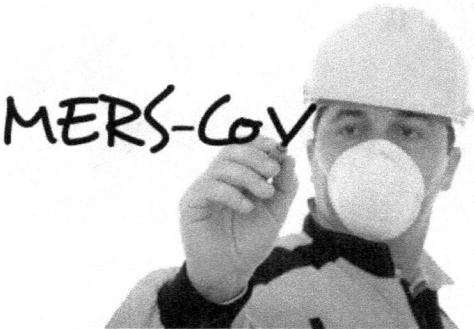

The Middle East Respiratory Syndrome Coronavirus (MERS-CoV) is slowly spreading through the Middle East and Asia. Transmission, so far, seems to happen when a close contact with an infected individual occurs. This type of transmission has led to many healthcare associated infections to this day. As an example, a patient that waited for 2.5 days in a Seoul emergency department, end it up transmitting the disease to 55 persons.

So far, the case-fatality rate is around 36 %, which is very high. However, this number may not be representative of a normal population and its kill rate is likely to be overestimated. A bias might exist when looking at the population who acquired the virus in Korea. Of the 171 cases, many had underlying medical conditions and had a median age of 55.

Ramblings about disinfection – Lalema inc.
Gaétan Lanthier & Rémi Charlebois

Official recommendations

CDC and Health Canada issued a few recommendations on infection control and prevention so far, and more is likely to be available soon. Regardless of their recommendations few data are available on environmental hygiene and disinfection practice regarding MERS-CoV in healthcare settings. Also, the transmission through the environment is not well known for this virus.

How to disinfect?

Regarding disinfection few information is available. Coronaviruses are non-enveloped virus which makes them more resistant to certain disinfectant. As an example, it is known that a 400 ppm solution of quaternary ammonium compounds is ineffective against those viruses. Sodium hypochlorite at a minimum of 1,000 ppm seems to be sufficient; however, a higher concentration would be optimal in healthcare settings. Very few data exist regarding other disinfectant technology.

At this moment, isolation with contact-droplets precaution is advised. In spite of the fact that it was suggested during the SARS outbreak that this type of isolation might not be sufficient. Even though these two viruses are similar, we must remember that many differences exist. Thus we must be careful with extrapolation of data.

Dilution is the Solution

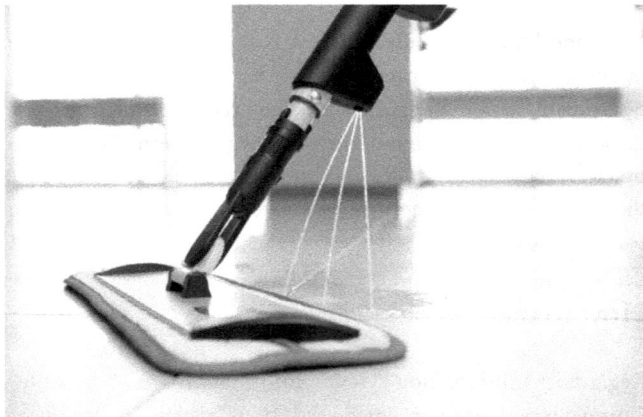

The dilution of chemical products in housekeeping is certainly one of the aspects where the lack of knowledge is most evident.

Dilution is often misunderstood

Effectively, there are unfortunately too many housekeepers that have the habit of adding a too large quantity of chemicals to their washing solution. Therefore, if they would come to a stop for an instant, in order to realize up to which point this may be harmful to their work, this bad habit would be lost very quickly.

We must indeed remember that cleaning chemical products are conceived to reach their maximum potential with a very precise volume of water.

Consequently, we must use a dilution measuring system that should be standardized for the whole working team.

Effects of under-dilution

With respect to Health and Safety, under dilution can cause:

- Dermatitis problems
- Respiratory tract problems
- Toxic fumes may cause cancer, difficult to prove and difficult to be recognized.

With respect to work efficiency and surfaces, under dilution can:

- Damage surfaces, since an under-diluted alkaline product will make a dull effect, by opening the pores of the floor coverings and thus allowing the deposit of alkalis. Acids, on the contrary, close the pores of the floor coverings and also burn the surface.
- Leave a film on the surface that will give a continuous streaky appearance and this film being greasy will facilitate the adherence of dirt.
- Cause enormous rinse problems because it will create foam in the solution container, which anyway has no cleaning effect.
- Disturb disinfection efficiency.
- Result in a loss of efficiency, since a well-diluted product reduces the physical demand to perform a task and favors the mechanical action.

Effects of over-dilution

Over dilution can cause:

- Result in no disinfection.
- Result in the loss of efficiency since an over-diluted product will increase the physical workload at the expense of the mechanical action.

The right dilution is always the best solution

The use of a dilution system does not have to be complicated or costly.

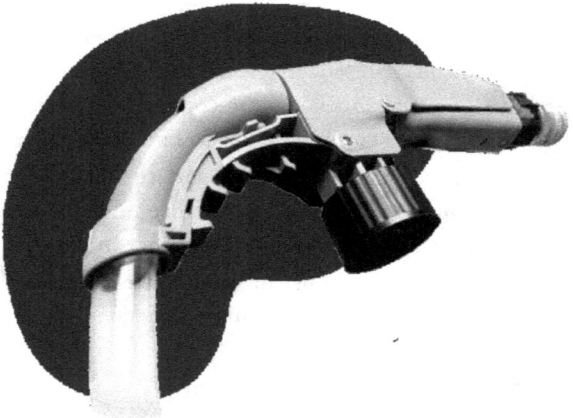

How to Reduce Fatigue and Nosocomial Infection at the Same Time

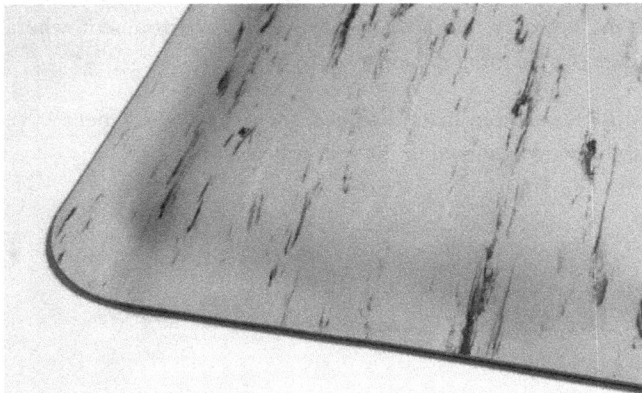

Working long hours in an upright position rings a bell to you? Back pain, stress and fatigue are your daily meals? There may be a solution for you.

First: Reduce fatigue with an anti-fatigue mat

One of the features found in this type of carpet is the presence of absorbent foam. Has it been developed by NASA? In fact, we only need to know if it works. If fatigue is reduced and comfort is improved, then risk of injury and error is reduced.

Second: a unique environment

Anti-fatigue mats are found in dry, wet or oily environment. It is, however, possible to have a dry environment where there is a risk of contamination.

Most ergonomic mats designed for a dry environment have no backing as shown in the following picture:

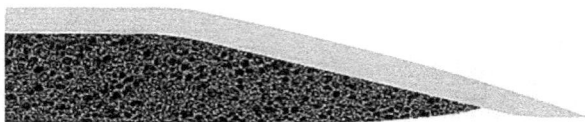

When the mat is placed in an environment where there is a risk of contamination, for example in an intensive care unit, a nurse workstation or an examination room, this can be a real problem. Indeed, how can one ensure the disinfection of such a foam pad, an absorbent material, is located under the carpet?

A suitable carpet for the Healthcare Environment

The solution? Get a sealed carpet.

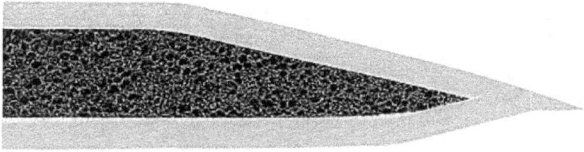

This type of carpet is an ergonomic mat designed specifically for critical areas in terms of infection control.

- Non-porous carpet completely sealed sides
- Resistant surface cuts and punctures
- Very easy to clean and disinfect
- Excellent anti-fatigue properties

Happy Global Handwashing Day

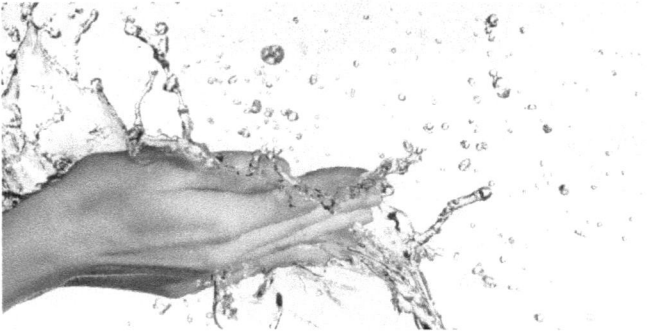

To increasing awareness and understanding let's talk about the importance of handwashing.

Handwashing is easy

Only a small amount of water and soap are necessary to accomplish a small action that provides great benefits. It takes 30 seconds and a bit of hand rubbing.

Handwashing works

Washing hands after using the toilet and before handling food can dramatically reduce the risk of infections such as foodborne infection. This year, handwashing was critical in the prevention of the Ebola virus in West Africa.

Ramblings about disinfection – Lalema inc.
Gaétan Lanthier & Rémi Charlebois

Handwashing is for everyone

We always ask children to wash their hands before eating, when they are back from school or after playing in the yard. From toddlers to elderly, handwashing never loses its importance. Infections can be transmitted by anyone to everyone. In order to protect children or elderly, everyone should wash their hands. After all, it is the most cost-effective public health intervention.

Ebola, How to Disinfect Surfaces

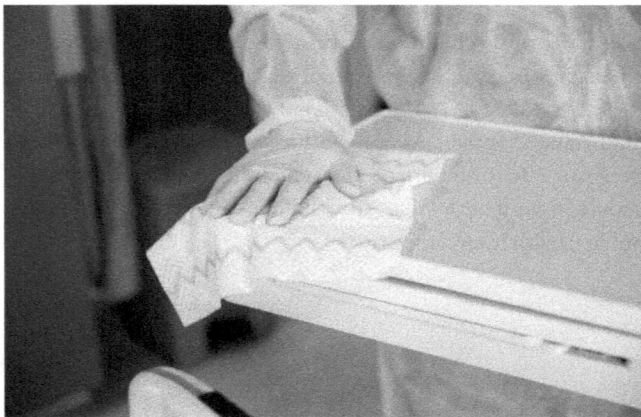

In 2014-2015, the Ebola outbreak in West Africa became an epidemic that spreaded beyond Africa. Although the risk of transmission is relatively low, it was the largest ever recorded outbreak of Ebola. WHO, CDC and other NGOs declared a state of emergency and fought tirelessly to limit the outbreak.

Importance of hygiene when it comes to Ebola

The debate today is polarized on the ethical use of experimental drugs. However, we noticed that few media state of the propagation modes and the importance of hygiene against this virus. Although transmission is being achieved mainly by direct contact between two people, contaminated objects and surfaces represent a risk that is hard to assess. Thus, the CDC and WHO suggest that objects in direct contact with the patient must be decontaminated properly and that medical or objects contaminated with body fluids must be incinerated.

Stabilized Sodium Hypochlorite

All well and good, but what product can be used to disinfect appropriately? Ebola Virus Outbreak Guidelines written by members of the Ministry of Public Health of Gabon suggest the use of sodium hypochlorite.

Ebola Virus, Are We Ready?

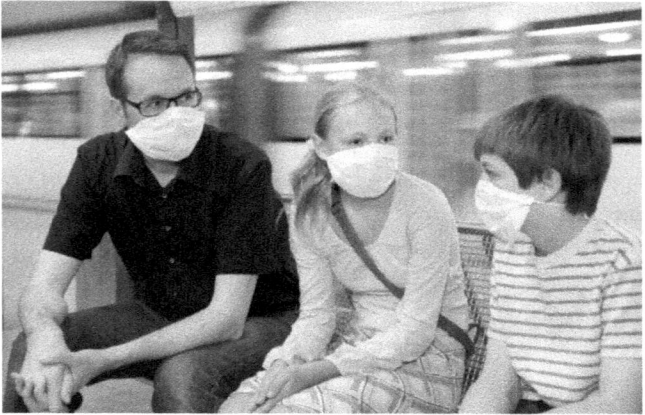

Are we ready to deal with a global pandemic of Ebola?

Western public health agencies are meant reassuring. Our hospitals are better equipped to deal with potential cases. The Quebec ministry of health issued a policy of transparency and now disclosed suspected cases in Quebec on its web site.

What to do to prevent the spread of Ebola virus in your institute?

Quebec Hospitals can refer to the official guide written by l'Institut national de santé publique du Québec. This fact sheet sets out the recommendations of the Comité sur les infections nosocomiales du Québec (CINQ) for Ebola virus disease prevention and control measures for Quebec hospitals.

- *Use a 5% bleach solution (sodium hypochlorite) with a concentration of 5000 ppm to disinfect surfaces or objects contaminated by blood or other body fluids.*

- *Use a 5000 ppm chlorine solution for the final disinfection.*

Disinfection is, therefore, more than ever critical to limit the spread of infection. The quality of the product is critical. Ebola is generally considered the world's most dangerous viruses. Might as well use the best disinfectant!

Robots to Destroy Ebola?

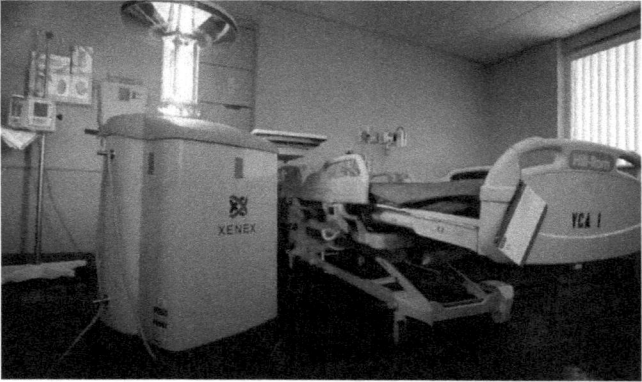

Robots are soldiers in a war against HAI's

Two Canadian hospitals have recently acquired a machine enabling surface disinfection in health institutions.

The Juravinksi hospital in Hamilton has started a year trial of a robot that costs $95,000 that burns the bacteria with UV rays. The general hospital of Vancouver has also started a trial of a UV robot that is 1.65 meters tall working with UV rays as well. The effectiveness of these machines relies on the properties of the UV rays, or rather on the xenon UV rays, to sterilize and kill microscopic contaminants.

Ebola outbreak

Recently, with the Ebola Outbreak, the Texas Health Presbyterian Hospital in Dallas, where 42-year-old Thomas

Eric Duncan, the first person to be diagnosed with Ebola in the USA, was being treated, also uses such device. But was it enough?

What about your hospital?

The goal of these robots is not to replace the housekeeping staff, nor the products employed for critical disinfections, but rather to complete their work, and to avoid that a single microscopic bacteria could take the life of a person whose immune system is weak.

Is your plan ready? Is your staff trained well enough? Do you have a stabilized chlorinated cleaner disinfectant in stock?

Ebola, How Does it Spread?

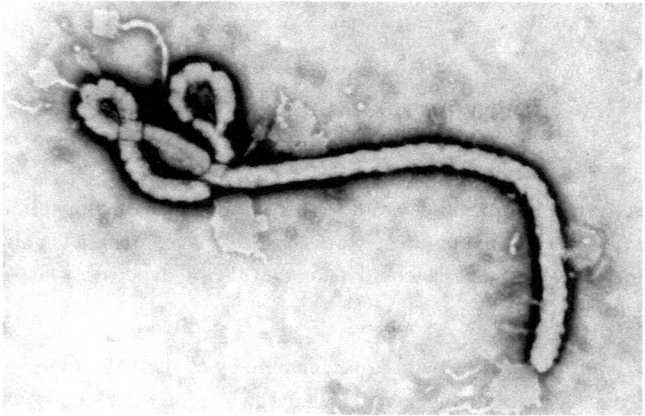

The Ebola Virus

Ebola is a virus. There is currently no vaccine or treatment. It causes severe disease, causing serious symptoms including vomiting and bleeding. The mortality rate can reach 90%. Primary infection comes from a contact with an infected animal and it can spread quickly.

How can you get infected with Ebola?

By coming into contact with bodily fluids such as blood, urine, feces and vomit. Also by one of the following means: by contact with a dead victim, by ingestion of infected animal meat or by having sexual intercourse with an infected person.

What are the symptoms of Ebola?

The symptoms of Ebola are fever, headache, nausea and fatigue. It may also include bleeding from nose, mouth or eyes, coughing, diarrhea or vomiting with the possible presence of blood.

How to prevent Ebola transmission

The risk of transmission of the Ebola virus in Canada is very low. However, certain precautions must be taken. The Public Health Agency of Canada also recommends that travelers avoid all nonessential travel to Guinea, Liberia and Sierra Leone.

There is a risk only if you have been in contact with sick people. In such case, if you experience symptoms, call 8-1-1 (Quebec) and inform them of your discomfort. You will be directed to the healthcare center care that can help you.

What to do to prevent the spread of Ebola virus

It is important that each healthcare center that can receive a potentially infectious patient put in place appropriate precautionary measures. Thus, it is important to have the required equipment for this type of care.

Zika Virus, Where Does It Come From?

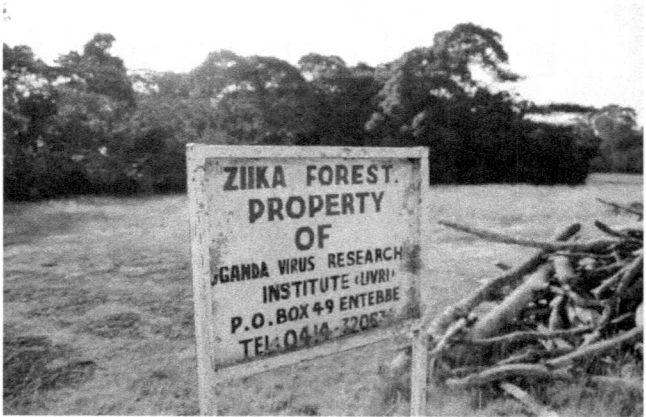

Everything started back in the 40s. A research team in Uganda, led by Alexander Haddow, was studying the yellow fever virus near Entebbe. In April 1950, the team isolated a new virus from a monkey used as a test animal in the Ziika forest.

The first human clinical case was described in 1954 in Nigeria. Then, in 1956, an experiment was conducted on a volunteer who got infected with the Zika virus through bites of infected mosquitoes. The subject developed a weak fever with a mild skin rash. The symptoms disappeared within a week. No more doubt, the Zika virus can infect human being via a mosquito bite.

The Zika virus was isolated in numerous species of *Aedes* mosquitoes in Africa and Malaysia. In 2007, the virus was identified in Micronesia, in what was the first large-scale epidemic. Since then, the Zika virus has been considered as an emerging virus.

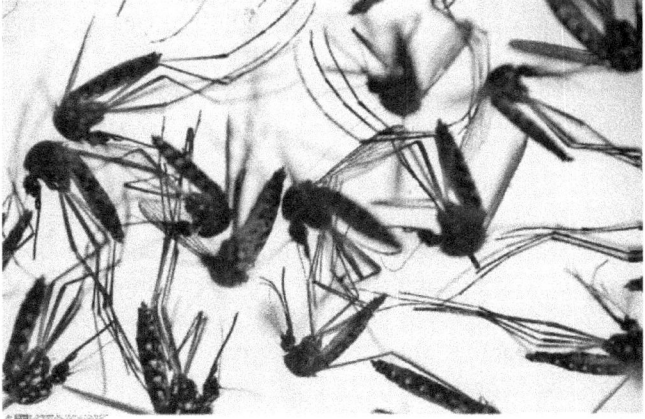

Aedes aegypti Mosquitoes

During 2013, an outbreak was raging in French Polynesia. The virus rapidly spread and was confirmed in the five archipelagos of French Polynesia which count roughly 270,000 inhabitants. Between October 2013 and March 2014, the number of infected persons is estimated at 28,000 individuals. 73 cases of Guillain-Barré syndrome were described during this epidemic. The Guillain-Barré syndrome is a rare affection that can cause muscle weakness and even paralysis. Sporadic cases of Zika virus disease were described throughout Oceania.

In Brazil, at the start of 2015, an increasing number of patients presenting symptoms similar to the Dengue virus disease were observed. This increase stroke the attention of Brazilian Public Health authorities. An infectious disease specialist evaluated some patients and laboratory results confirmed that the virus neither the Dengue nor the Chikungunya virus. In March 2015, the Zika virus was confirmed by the Carlos Chagas Institute. It was the first time that Zika virus disease was contracted in the Americas.

The virus strain isolated in Brazil is somewhat close to the Asian strains with similarities to the virus isolated in Oceania a few years ago. Some experts believe that the virus was imported into Brazil during the World Championship of pirogue (va'a) that was held in Brazil in August 2014. Four Oceanian countries where the virus is circulating were present at the Championship.

To this day, it was estimated that about 1.5 million cases of Zika virus disease occurred in Brazil, which makes it the biggest Zika virus outbreak ever recorded. It is now spreading to other countries where the *Aedes* mosquitoes are present.

The Zika virus is suspected to be linked to microcephaly touching the fetus of infected mothers. According to the Brazil Health Minister, 4,783 suspected cases of microcephaly were described so far (February 2016). Active research is ongoing to find if and how can the Zika virus be related to birth defects.

Ramblings about disinfection – Lalema inc.
Gaétan Lanthier & Rémi Charlebois

Zika Virus is there a Risk for Surface Contamination?

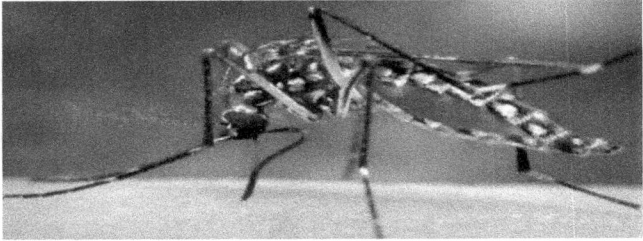

Zika virus is an arbovirus transmitted by *Aedes* mosquitoes. It was discovered in 1947 in a monkey in Uganda. Zika virus is mainly present in Central America and South America but also in Africa and Oceania.

Zika virus, what is it?

With the Zika virus, it is reported that nearly 3 out of 4 infections do not present any symptoms. When symptoms occur, it looks like the flu: fever, headache, body aches with rashes, beginning 3-12 days after being bitten by mosquitoes. Zika virus can also manifest as conjunctivitis or pain behind the eyes, as well as swelling of the hands or feet. The disease is not directly fatal.

Why are pregnant women particularly at risk?

If a pregnant woman is infected, she can pass the virus to her baby through the placenta or during birth.

It is suspected that pregnant women infected with the virus could give birth to babies with microcephaly. Babies are born with a head circumference below 33 cm and irreversible mental retardation.

However, there is no fully proven causal link between Zika and microcephaly and because some mothers do not believe they had the virus.

What precautions should you take?

There is no vaccine against the Zika virus. It is recommended to protect yourself against bites by wearing long clothing and using insect repellent and mosquito nets. According to the official website of the Government of Canada (canadaensante.gc.ca)

No local transmission of Zika virus has been reported in Canada. At present, the mosquitoes that transmit Zika virus are not found in Canada because of the climate. So the likelihood of transmission is very low in the country.

Low potential for contamination of surfaces

Zika virus is mainly transmitted through mosquito bites. However, hygiene and safety should follow their normal procedures including disinfection of high potential contamination of surfaces and hand washing.

Why Choose a Ready-to-use Bleach Based Cleaner-Disinfectant?

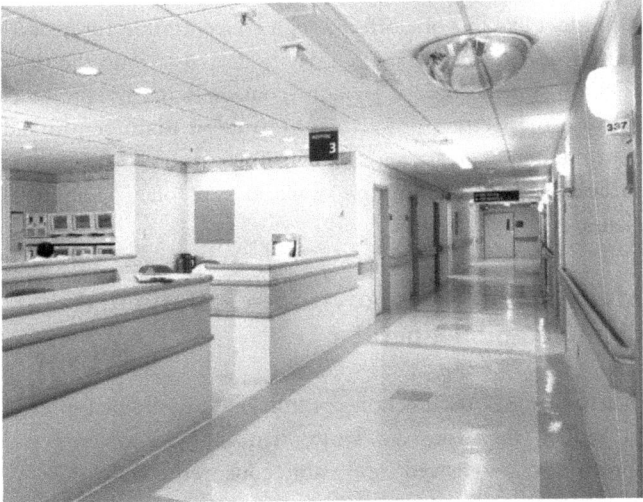

In the actual market, you can find many cleaner-disinfectants. When it comes to consumer products, you'll find a lot of brands, most of them are ready to use. It means you do not have to dilute the product and use it as is to disinfect. For industrial and institutional use, most of cleaner-disinfectants are concentrated if not ultra-concentrated. In that case, why choose a ready-to-use Bleach based Cleaner-Disinfectant for institutional use?

Main benefit of a low-foam concentrated product

A product like this one offers a high concentration for general disinfection in hospitals. On a day to day basis, with the right dilution system, the surfactants contained in the products increase the wetting power of **chlorinated disinfectant** and contribute to degrease and remove dirt from hard non-porous surfaces such as countertops, walls, floors, toilets, commode chairs, etc.

Main benefit of a ready-to-use chlorinated disinfectant cleaner

When it comes to infection control, one important aspect is to reduce the risk. We know that dilution systems can sometimes be flawed and not consistent with delivery concentration. Therefore, it is crucial to obtain a consistent known concentration.

Of course, it may generate more plastic in the environment. Recycling may then be on option to consider. At the same time, when patient's lives are at risk, all factors that can reduce the risk is of important value.

Ramblings about disinfection – Lalema inc.
Gaétan Lanthier & Rémi Charlebois

www.ingramcontent.com/pod-product-compliance
Lightning Source LLC
Chambersburg PA
CBHW061840220326
41599CB00027B/5354